FIRST AID GUIDES.

Basic First Aid Objectives And Procedures.

Saint Dowell

Table of contents

INTRODUCTION

Every time could be a bad time for you or people close to you to get sick or hurt. Using simple first aid techniques may help you stop a minor accident from getting worse. In a severe medical crisis, you might even save a life.

Determining the principles of first aid is essential because of this. If you want to build on the information you learn from this article, think about taking a first aid course. First aid education is offered by numerous companies.

In an emergency, injuries are essentially a given. There is a danger that whatever is producing the emergency will harm you; for example, you might get burned in a fire or hit by falling debris during an earthquake. But during the panic, injuries are also sustained.

The Meaning Of First Aid.

Giving someone who has become suddenly ill or injured first aid is the procedure of providing basic medical care.

When someone is experiencing a medical emergency, first aid can refer to the initial care that is offered to them.

They might be able to survive with this support's assistance until rescue arrives.

In other instances, first aid refers to the treatment of a small injury. For instance, minor burns, wounds, and insect stings can frequently be treated with just first aid.

Rather than treating patients, its main objective is to offer emergency aid to a sick or injured individual there and then. First aid can prevent the problem from getting worse while you wait for more thorough medical care.

Five Primary Goals Of First Aid.

- protect life.
- Stop a disease or injury from getting worse.
- Encourage healing.
- alleviate the agony.
- safeguard the unconscious.

The protection of life.

In a first aid course, life preservation scenarios include administering CPR or attending to someone who is choking. The prevention of additional serious illnesses, such as brain damage and even a heart attack, which can occur in a matter of minutes, is achieved by maintaining air circulation in the body and opening up obstructed airways while awaiting medical assistance.

Stop an illness or injury from getting worse.

As part of first aid training, you will learn how to treat wounds and injuries to prevent further harm or spread.

For instance, if the patient is bleeding, the first responder should try to control the bleeding until expert medical assistance comes.

Encouraging healing.

Using a first aid kit to assist the individual in need is part of promoting healing. This could entail cleaning, sanitizing, and bandaging a wound. An antibiotic ointment may occasionally be applied to aid in the healing process.

Pain management.

Only if there are no risks to the patient should one consider providing pain treatment. It is not advised to administer painkillers if the patient is bleeding. It's better to consult a medical professional before prescribing any kind of drug.

Safeguard the unconscious.
A safe evacuation from a hazardous area, such as a fire or busy road, to a location where they are safer, is part of protecting someone unconscious. Participants in first aid training are taught how to position a person who is unconscious to prevent obstruction of the breathing airways. Assuring someone's safety when they are unconscious is the main objective of protecting them.

CHAPTER ONE

Keep In Mind The "Three Ps."

Before offering assistance, make sure the area is safe.

Use mild pressure, a disinfectant, and bandages to treat wounds and scrapes.

Use ice, compression, and elevation to the limb as needed to treat sprains.

Make use of cool liquids, cool clothing, and shade to alleviate heat exhaustion.

Use warm liquids and a warm covering to treat hypothermia.

Determine the nature and degree of the burn before treating it. To stop infection, drape a loose cloth over the wound.

Use a cold pack and maintain stability and immobilization of the broken area to treat fractures.

If someone who has been hurt stops breathing, perform CPR.

Initial Care

You must memorize these 10 principles.
Even if you are not hurt, you can come
across someone who is and needs medical
attention.

Always make an effort to get injured people
medical attention from a professional. When
first responders are not immediately
accessible during an emergency, try your
best to give the best care you can until help
arrives. Do your best to get the injured
individual to qualified caregivers, but keep
in mind that major injuries always require
more advanced care.

But even these basic first aid techniques can
make a big difference in helping someone
who has been hurt. All you need to do is use
a few supplies from your survival kit
properly.

First, the "Three Ps"

The main aims of first aid are known as the "Three P's." As follows:

- keep life alive.
- avert future harm.
- Encourage recovery.

The simplicity of these objectives may seem excessive, but it is on purpose. It's all too easy to panic when someone is hurt and forget what you need to do to help. The Three s serve as a helpful reminder of the fundamentals: do everything you can to save the person's life; try to prevent them from suffering additional injuries; and try to aid in their healing.

CHAPTER TWO

Examine The Environment For Hazards.

It's necessary to look around the area for any dangers before offering aid to someone who is hurt. A self-inflicted injury is something you don't desire. This is not an insensitive safety measure. The simple truth is that if you hurt yourself, you can't help someone else who's hurt. To avoid getting hurt, take some time to survey the environment before rushing to assist someone.

A severe storm can be occurring outside, for instance, and you might see someone who is hurt and unable to get inside shelter outside. Search for dangers before you sprint outside to assist them. Objects being thrown by strong winds Do any trees or buildings look particularly

After evaluating these risks, you may more effectively plan how to approach and rescue the injured person.

CHAPTER THREE

Handling Scrapes And Cuts.

Our bodies need blood to function.
When someone is bleeding, you want to stop
as much blood from leaving their body as
you can.
Try to locate a fresh bandage or towel. Then,
20 to 30 minutes of light pressure should be
applied.
Gently run clean water over the wound to
clean it. Keep soap away from an exposed
wound.
On the wound, apply an antibiotic such as
Neosporin.

Bandage the wound after cleaning it.
Ask the person bleeding from the nose to
lean forward. Once the blood flow has
stopped, press a towel across the nostrils.

The body often heals minor wounds and scrapes extremely quickly. But, more serious wounds could need medical attention. Having severe wounds:

CHAPTER FOUR

Put Pressure On.

Apply no ointments. To stop pollutants from infecting the wound, cover the region with a loose towel.
Immediately seek medical attention.
Treatment of Sprains;
Sprains are typically minor ailments that heal on their own the majority of the time. Yet you can take action to reduce the swelling. A wounded area's blood flow is what causes swelling. Using ice can help with edema reduction. The blood arteries are constricted by ice, which lowers blood flow.

CHAPTER FIVE

Elevate The Limb That Is Damaged, And Place The Wounded Area With Ice.

Avoid putting ice on the skin directly. Put the object in a cloth bag or a plastic bag with ice.

Compress the wounded area while you heal, Wrap it securely or place it in a brace.

To inhibit circulation, avoid wrapping it too tightly,

Ice for some time.

Finally, condense repeatedly.

Make sure the victim refrains from putting any weight on the hurt limb.

CHAPTER SIX

Treatment For Heat Exhaustion.

Long-term exposure to high temperatures can lead to heat exhaustion, especially if the person is engaging in strenuous activity or hasn't taken enough water. Heat exhaustion signs and symptoms include;

- chilly and wet skin.
- heavy perspiration.
- Dizziness.
- poor pulse.
- muscle pain.
- Nausea and Headaches.

For the treatment of heat exhaustion:

Bring the person somewhere shaded and out of the sun,
Keep the person covered by any things that can block sunlight if there are no shaded areas nearby,
Keep the person hydrated by providing water,

To bring down their body temperature, use a cool towel on their forehead.

CHAPTER SEVEN

Treating Hypothermia.

Hypothermia can develop after prolonged exposure to low temperatures.
As your body temperature falls below 95 degrees Fahrenheit, it starts to happen.

Hypothermia signs include:

- Shivering.
- murmured words or speech.
- Weekend pulse.
- Coordination issues.
- Confusion.
- chilly, rosy skin.
- consciousness loss.
- Hypothermia therapy.

Be kind to the individual who is ill. Avoid rubbing them or moving them too abruptly, doing so could cause a cardiac attack.

Remove any wet clothing and take the victim out of the cold.

Use heat packs while draping blankets over the person. Applying heat directly to the skin should be avoided as this could seriously harm the skin.

Provide warm liquids to the patient. Remember that the ground could be a source of cold if you place the person there. Lay warm materials on the surface that the person will be lying on.

CHAPTER EIGHT

Burns Treatments.

It is important to determine the type and degree of the burn before beginning treatment. There are four varieties.
Just the outermost layers of the skin are harmed by first-degree burns.

The skin is swollen, and red, and has a sunburn-like appearance.
Second-degree burn: The skin's innermost layer has some burn damage. Watch out for swelling and blistered skin. This kind of burn typically causes excruciating pain.
Burn of the third degree: The entire inner layer of skin has been burned. The damage is either white or has a darker color.
 Some third-degree burns are so severe that because the nerve endings have been damaged, there may not even be any pain.

Burns of the fourth degree: have reached the tendons and bones after permeating all surrounding tissues.
There are also two different levels of burn severity: a minor burn and a large burn.

First-degree burns and light second-degree burns are minor burns.
a severe burn.

Apply cool water to the affected region (avoid icy or very cold water).
Keep your blisters intact.
Using aloe vera as a moisturizer, cover the region.
Remove the injured person from direct sunlight.
Ibuprofen or acetaminophen should be administered to the burn victim to ease their pain.
Significant burns are very serious wounds that call for medical attention. For assistance with a severe burn victim:

Use no creams or ointments.
To stop pollutants from infecting the
wound, cover it with loose materials.

CHAPTER NINE

Allergic Responses.

Your body will have allergic reactions if it is overly sensitive to a foreign chemical. Allergies can result from bee stings, particular foods, or medicine components. Any of the aforementioned allergens are capable of causing the potentially fatal allergic reaction known as anaphylaxis.

Using an EpiPen is the best method to handle an allergic response. A small, ergonomic needle called an EpiPen is used to provide epinephrine (adrenaline) to someone who is having a severe allergic response. The effects of the allergic reaction are typically reduced with epinephrine.

If someone is having an allergic reaction:

Keep the person at peace, Inquire whether they carry an EpiPen with them and utilize one.

The individual should lie on their back.

Keep their feet 12 inches off the ground.

Make sure the person is wearing loose clothing so they can breathe.

Give them no food, drink, or medication.

Use an EpiPen if necessary. Find out how to administer an EpiPen to someone experiencing a response.

After using an EpiPen, wait 5–15 minutes.

CHAPTER TEN

Fracture Care.

When someone suffers a bone fracture, it can often be extremely simple to tell. Although occasionally it's not. Detecting a fracture in a person begins with:

You shouldn't attempt to straighten a broken limb.
To stabilize and stop the region from moving, use cushioning or a splint.
Wrap the region in a cold compress. Never put it on your skin directly. With a plastic bag or a cloth, wrap it up.
As much as you can, keep the area raised.
Ibuprofen or another NSAID should be administered to the patient.

CPR is performed in 10.

Cardiopulmonary resuscitation is known by the acronym CPR. An unresponsive person might be given CPR to help them breathe and get the blood flowing again. The life-saving technique of CPR is very significant. Nonetheless, becoming familiar with CPR is a heart attack first aid.

Call 911 if you believe someone may be having a heart attack. Help them find and take the nitroglycerin if it has been prescribed to them. As soon as medical assistance is on the way, wrap them in a blanket and give them comfort.

CHAPTER ELEVEN

Equip Yourself With The Proper Equipment.

The aforementioned techniques are simple to use and don't require medical knowledge, yet they have the power to save lives and shield those who have been hurt from suffering severe wounds or infections. Ensure that your supply of survival supplies contains a first aid kit, and remember to replenish it annually as its materials run out or expire.

CHAPTER TWELVE

First Aid Kits On Infants.

It's a good idea to carry a fully stocked first aid kit in your home and car to be ready for unforeseen emergencies. Making your first aid kit is also an option.

If you have a baby, you might need to swap out or add infant-friendly options for some of the supplies in a typical first aid kit. For illustration, a baby thermometer and baby acetaminophen or ibuprofen should be included in your kit.

Also, it's crucial to keep the equipment out of your baby's reach.

For further information on infant-friendly first aid, consult your pediatrician or primary care physician.

Standard first aid supplies ought to contain;

- various size adhesive bandages.
- numerous sizes of roller bandages.
- compress dressings that absorb.
- sterile tissues.
- sticky cloth tape.
- three-sided bandages.
- sanitizing wipes.
- antibiotic cream, ibuprofen, acetaminophen, or aspirin.
- Calamine lotion, hydrocortisone cream, and vinyl or nitrile gloves.
- security pins.
- scissors.
- tweezers.
- thermometer, breathing mask, and quick cold pack.

Moreover, it's a good idea to include a list of your doctors, emergency contacts, and prescription medication in your first aid supplies.

CHAPTER THIRTEEN

Treatment For Bleeding Wounds.

Calling an ambulance and then stopping the bleeding as quickly as feasible should be a first aid provider's top priority when a person is suffering from severe bleeding.

This can be accomplished by applying pressure to the wound using a clean dressing for wounds without any embedded objects. After the bleeding stops, the wound needs to be dressed with a fresh, clean dressing.

CHAPTER FOURTEEN

First Aiding Drowning.

The priority is to rescue anyone who is found drowning or struggling in the water. Always make sure it is safe to do so before diving in if this calls for it.

Call 911 to send an ambulance as soon as the individual reaches the shore, and make sure they are breathing. If they are, their head should be positioned lower than their body in the recovery position; if not, CPR must be performed along with five rescue breaths.

CHAPTER FIFTEEN

Treatment Of An Electrical Jolt.

To prevent further contact between an electric shock victim and the electrical supply, the power at the mains must be turned off.

If the person is not breathing after the power has been turned off, an ambulance needs to be contacted right away. Otherwise, medical attention should be sought to ensure that they do not have any other wounds.

CHAPTER SIXTEEN

Poisoning First Aid.

A person becomes poisoned when they are exposed to material that harms their health. When a person has been poisoned, an ambulance must be called, and the paramedics must be informed of the poison's identity if known.

Treatment for poisoning is challenging since its effects might change based on the material to which a person has been exposed. However, to prevent poisoning someone else, the person shouldn't be compelled to vomit, and if CPR needs to be started, they shouldn't be given rescue breaths.

CHAPTER SEVENTEEN

First Aiding Shock.

Insufficiently oxygenated blood inhibits important organs from receiving oxygen, resulting in shock. Because of this, someone in shock has to be taken to the hospital in an ambulance. Also, they should be provided a coat or blanket to keep warm and should be laid out with their feet elevated. Never give food or drink to someone who is in shock.

CHAPTER EIGHTEEN

First Aiding Stroke.

To lessen the effects of a stroke on a person's life, they must receive emergency care as quickly as possible.

The following are some signs of a stroke:

Face: One side of their face can have drooped.
Arms: They can be unable to raise one or both arms or maintain their elevation.
Speech: It could be hard to understand them or their speech is slurred.
An ambulance must be called if a person exhibits any of these symptoms.

A person must successfully finish relevant workplace first aid training before serving as a first aider.

CHAPTER NINETEEN

Aiding Blisters.

Skin injury is protected by blisters while it heals.

Some blisters require treatment, while others do not. The severity of the blister and your general health will determine if you need to treat it.

A Blood Blister: What Is It?
Steps to Take.
It is better to ignore a blister if it is small, closed, and painless. To avoid rubbing, which can cause it to enlarge and explode, you might cover it.

Avoid popping blisters because doing so could allow bacteria to enter the wound and lead to an infection.

For this more serious blister treatments, use these first aid instructions:

- Do a hand wash.
- At the blister's edge, drill a few tiny holes.
- Push the fluid away gently.
- Put on some antibiotic cream.
- Apply a bandage.
- Prevent further rubbing or pressure on the area if at all feasible.

You should avoid self-blister draining if you have a weakened immune system since you are more susceptible to infection.
However, to assist avoid infection, your doctor can decide to drain it.

When a blister spontaneously ruptures,
- Use only clean water to gently cleanse the area.
- Cover the skin flap with a gentle hand.

Unless it is filthy, torn, or there is pus
underneath it, smooth the flap of damaged
skin over the freshly exposed skin.
smear it with petroleum jelly.
Put a bandage over it.
Every time it gets wet, change the bandage.
As you go to bed, take it off to allow the
space to air out.

CHAPTER TWENTY

First Treatment for Nosebleeds.

Digital trauma, more often known as picking
your nose, is the most frequent cause of
nosebleeds.

Other reasons for a bloody nose include:

- Chilly or warm air.
- The nasal passages are irritated by
  chemical smells.
- influenza and allergies.
- blowing your nose too forcefully or too
  often

injuries to the nose.

- distorted septum (crooked nasal
  cartilage).

Nasal polyps or nasal tumors are growths in
the nasal canal and sinuses that can be
malignant or non-cancerous bleeding
conditions, such as hemophilia and
leukemia.

In other cases, a person may just need that kind of care. In other instances, administering first aid is a way to keep someone alive and stop their condition from growing worse until paramedics arrive or until they are sent to the hospital.

The best way to prepare for these circumstances is to take proper first aid training.

ABCs of First Aids.

Airways: The person's airway should be your priority if they are having trouble breathing.

Breathing:Provide rescue breathing if someone is still not breathing after you have opened up their airway.

Circulation: Use chest compressions while performing rescue breathing to keep the victim's blood flowing. Check the pulse of someone who is breathing but not moving. Chest compressions should be given if their heart has stopped.

The ABCs can be expressed more simply as:

Awake: Try to wake up the person if they aren't awake. Continue to the following step if they don't awaken, and make sure someone is dialing 911.
Breathing?:start rescue breathing and chest compressions if the person is unconscious and not breathing. then advance to the following;

Take care as you normally would: Follow the 911 operator's instructions or carry on providing care until an ambulance comes when you call for assistance.

Several first aid training programs additionally include D and E:

D may stand for an automated external defibrillator, disability evaluation, or life-threatening hemorrhage (AED).
An AED is a machine that shocks the heart to get it to begin beating once more. E can mean; Examining the person for symptoms of an injury, hemorrhage, allergies, or other issues after confirming that they are breathing and their heart is beating.

Where You Can Learn First Aid.

You can learn how to perform chest compressions, perform rescue breathing, and use an AED by enrolling in a formal CPR course. You can find training through the American Red Cross, the first responders in your neighborhood, and online.

Many public spaces and commercial establishments have AEDs. Even if you have

no experience, these first aid tools are
designed to be simple to use.

CHAPTER TWENTY-ONE

Bleeding First Aid.

There are some fundamentals about how blood functions that you should be aware of in case someone is hurt and bleeding.

You can determine the severity of the injury by observing the color and movement of the blood as it leaves the body:

Capillaries: The smallest blood vessels, or capillaries, are where bleeding appears to trickle. Typically, bleeding of this type will stop on its own.

Veins: Blood that flows steadily and has a dark red color is probably coming from the veins. This kind of bleeding can range in intensity from mild to severe.
The arteries are the biggest blood vessels and the ones that transport the most

oxygen. If they are harmed, they will bleed brilliant red.

With this type of bleeding, blood loss can happen very quickly.

With first aid, almost all bleeding can be stopped. A person may go into shock and maybe pass away if excessive bleeding continues.

CHAPTER TWENTY-TWO

Acute Puncture Wound Care.

If you have disposable gloves, put them on or wash your hands. You will be shielded from contagious illnesses transferred by blood, such as HIV/AIDS and viral hepatitis.

- Water-rinse the injury,
- Dress the wound in gauze or a rag (e.g., towel, blanket, clothing).
- Use direct pressure to halt the blood flow and promote coagulation (when blood naturally thickens to stop blood loss).
- If you can, raise the area of the person's body that is bleeding above their head.
- If the cloth gets wet, leave it in place. More blood will be lost if the top layer is removed since it will prevent the blood from clotting properly. Change it and, if necessary, add more levels.

- A fresh bandage should be applied to the wound once the bleeding has ceased.

Speak with a doctor if it is a serious wound.
Wide side separations can be seen in the wound.
After applying pressure, the wound begins to seep blood.

An animal or person bite caused the damage.
The damage is a burn, electrical, or puncture wound.
You believe that there is arterial bleeding.
The bandages are dripping with blood.
Bleeding has not stopped, a second person who can continue providing first aid as you drive should be present if you are driving the patient to the hospital.

CHAPTER TWENTY-THREE

Choking First Aid.

When something, such as food, blocks a person's trachea, they can choke. It's a serious incident that could result in loss of consciousness or even death.

Choking symptoms include:

- wheezing, gasping, or gagging.
- lack of ability to speak or create noise.
- bluish-greening of the face.
- taking hold of the throat.
- arm motions.
- Looking anxious.

Doing the Heimlich Maneuver,
A sequence of abdominal thrusts known as the Heimlich maneuver can be used to free someone who is choking. Only use this first aid procedure if the person is indeed choking.

Before taking any action, inquire as to whether the person is choking. Always keep in mind that if someone is talking or coughing, they are not choking.

These are the actions:

- Lean the person forward while standing behind them.
- Encircle their waist with your arms.
- Put your clenched hand between their ribcage and navel (belly button).
- With the other hand, grab your fist.
- In five rapid thrusts under the target's ribcage, thrust your clenched hand hard backward and upward.
- Continue until the thing comes up in a cough.
- If the person is overweight or pregnant, do the thrusts about the chest rather than the abdomen.

If someone is unconscious while they are
choking:

- Kneel over them and place them on
  their back.
- Just above their belly button, place the
  heel of your hand.
- Stack it with your other hand on top.
- To move the item, do fast upward
  thrusts.

CHAPTER TWENTY-FOUR

Aiding a Child Who Is Choking.

Start with back strikes if a baby is choking:

Baby should be placed face down across
your forearm.
They can be supported on your lap or upper
thigh.
With their head pointing down and lower
than their torso, hold their chest in one
hand and their jaw in the other.
Give the infant five sharp, hard punches to
the back between the shoulder blades with
the heel of your free hand.
Try chest thrusts if back blows are
unsuccessful:

- As you turn the infant around, support
  them by holding them on your lap.
- Hold the back of their head with one
  hand while keeping it angled

downward and lower than their torso
to keep it steady.

- Organize your fingers into a two or
  three-finger grid immediately below
  the nipples on the baby's chest.
- Five fast downward thrusts will push
  the breastbone in approximately 1.5
  inches.
- You might need to do CPR on an
  unconscious infant who is choking
  until emergency aid comes.

CONCLUSION

In Conclusion, when giving first aid, it's crucial to safeguard yourself from infectious diseases and other dangers.
To better safeguard yourself, Before approaching an ill or injured individual, always look out for any dangers to your safety.
Keep your distance from bodily fluids like blood, vomit, and others.
Use safety gear when doing rescue breathing or treating someone with an open wound, such as nitrile or vinyl gloves or a breathing barrier.
Wash your hands with soap and water right after giving first aid
Basic first aid frequently prevents a minor problem from going worse. The provision of first aid in a medical emergency may even save a life. Someone should undergo treatment if they have a severe injury or ailment.